Herbal Medicinal Remedies & Cleanses Made Easy

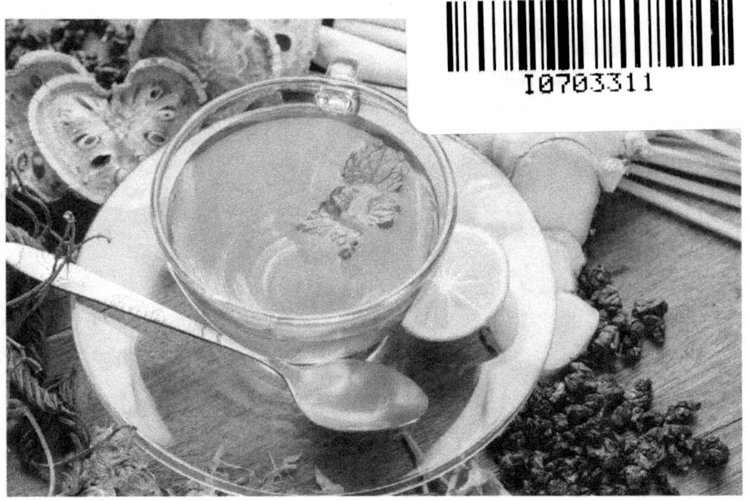

NATURE'S SUNSHINE PRODUCTS
1-800-233-8225

For wholesale price:

www.naturessunshine.com?
referrer=813321&offer=NSP

FOR BULK HERBS:
MOUNTAINROSEHERBS.COM

Outside of trauma, sickness and diseases are the results of the violation of the laws of nature, intentional or not. Germs do not cause disease, rather, pathogens proliferate when the environment is conducive to their growth.

Through the major channels of elimination (liver, lungs, lymph, kidneys, colon, skin), the body is assisted by bringing about and maintaining a healthy environment as toxins and poisons are eliminated (cleansing and detoxification). Building its nutritional reserves will keep bacteria, viruses, fungi, etc. from overstepping their boundaries, so to speak.

The body gives many signs that it's time to cleanse (headaches, lethargic, stiff joints, sinuses, allergies, acne, ulcers, skin problems, constipation, chronic diseases, and so on). When the toxic load is eliminated, skin is clearer, increased energy, thinking is clearer and symptoms are reduced, etc.

Herbs have been used for thousands of

years in the everyday lives of our ancestors. The herbal remedies and cleanses given in this booklet are for informational purposes. Please consult with your health practitioner.

In general, anytime is a good time to cleanse, but there are optimal times based on the seasons and phases of the moon (its magnetic connection with earth and everything on it, including us) to reap maximum benefits.

Spring and Autumn are the best times to do a long fast (anywhere from 7-21 days depending on which season). Summer and Winter are best for shorter fasts (anywhere from 1-7 days).

The new moon (completely dark and fully round) phase is a great time for new beginnings. It's when you have the greatest capacity to stick with a fast, break old habits and introduce new ones. Surgeries are best tolerated and less complications, etc.).

The waxing moon (going from dark to a light crescent) is a wonderful time to build up the body (strengthen, store energy, regenerate, rest, recover). It is an absorbing time (retain weight more easily, absorb nutrients). This is not a good time for surgeries; healing is slower and tendency for more scar tissue.

The full moon (completely round and fully

lit) is a phase when 1 or 2-day fasts are very effective. Things tend to reach their full capacity; more babies are born. There is a greater chance of bleeding out for surgeries during this phase and more complications. Water retention is also at its highest capacity.

The waning moon (going from light to a dark crescent) is a great time to start detoxing. It's a drying up time; less water retention. Weight is not gained as quickly even though more is eaten.

Note: Incorporate supplemental fiber and herbal cleansing teas daily during cleanses.

Mix fiber in water (psyllium husk, psyllium powder, chia seeds, slippery elm powder – shake vigorously and drink right away).

Cascara Sagrada, barberry, dandelion, fennel, fenugreek – make tea of one or more and add fresh lemon juice.

Be sure to prepare your body a couple days before your cleanse by eating light foods and eliminating dense, rich foods (no meats, processed foods or sugary food/drinks).

Of course, there are times of emergency when fasting is necessary, regardless of the season or phase. Also, stay warm since you can become colder than usually when fasting.

CLEANSES

The Seneca Indian Fast/Diet

From the Seneca Indians – In the book, "Good Health Through Diets" by Hanna Kroeger

This is a 4-day program and can be extended to 8 or 12 days by repeating. It is gently, simply and easy for the cleanser. This is also a "a "cleanse and build" for the body.

On the first day, the colon is cleansed. Second day, toxins, salts and excessive calcium deposits in the muscles, tissues and organs are released. Third day, the digestive tract is supplied with healthful, mineral rich bulk. The fourth day, the blood, lymph and organs are mineralized.

1st Day – Eat all the fruit you want (apples, berries, watermelon, pears, cherries), but not bananas or dried fruit. Diluted prune juice is also acceptable.

2nd Day – Drink all the herb teas you want (Chamomile, Raspberry, Spearmint, Hyssop). Bitters stimulate the digestive system.

3rd Day – Eat all the vegetable you want; raw or steamed or both.

4th Day – Make a pan of vegetable broth with whatever you have on hand (cabbage, onions, green peppers, parsley, etc. – season with herbs and Kelp if desired. Drink **only** the rich mineral **broth** all day.

The Master Cleanse (By Stanley Burroughs)

Purpose

- To dissolve and eliminate toxins and congestion.
- To cleanse the kidneys and digestive system.
- To purify the glands and cells.
- To eliminate all unusable waste and hardened material in the joints and muscles.
- To relieve pressure and irritation in the nerves, arteries and blood vessels.
- To build a healthy blood stream and keep youth and elasticity regardless of your years.

When to Use

- When sickness has developed (acute & chronic conditions).
- When digestive system needs rest and cleansing.
- When overweight has become a problem.
- When better assimilation and building of body tissue is needed.

How Often

- Cleanse for a minimum of 10 days to 40 days
- Cleanse has all the nutrition needed during this time.
- Three to four times a year will keep the body in a normal healthy condition.

How to Make

- 2 Tbsp. lemon or lime juice (about ½ lemon)
- 2 Tbsp. genuine Grade B maple syrup
- 1/10 cayenne pepper (type A blood use ginger)
- 10 ounces of medium hot water (spring or purified)

Maple syrup has a wide variety of minerals and vitamins (Sodium, Potassium, Calcium, Magnesium, Iron, Manganese, Copper, Phosphorus, Sulfur Silicon, Vitamin A, B1, B2, B6, C and B5. (Aguirre & Baker, 2016)

<u>Diabetics,</u> consult with your natural health practitioner for adjustments before undertaking this cleanse.

How Much to Drink

- Take six to twelve glasses daily during waking hours. No other food should be taken during the period of this cleanse. As you get hungry, drink another glass.
- Extra water may be taken. Mint tea may be taken <u>occasionally</u> for a change is taste.

Internal Salt Bath may be taken each morning of cleanse. Mix one quart warm water and two leveled teaspoons of non-iodized "Real Salt" sea salt. Drink entire quart first thing in the morning on an empty stomach. The entire digestive tract will be washed within one hour and several eliminations will likely occur. If no elimination, body was dehydrated and cells absorbed entire fluid.

How to Break This Fast

- For the first two days after fast, drink several 8-ounce glasses of fresh squeezed

> orange or pineapple juice during the day, as desired – drink slowly. This prepares the digestive system for assimilating regular food.
> - On the 3rd day, drink orange or pineapple juice in the morning. Eat raw fruit for lunch. Fruit or raw vegetable salad at night.
> - On 4th day, you are ready to eat normally.

If all this seems too hard, do it along with your regular eating, to start, then try one day and go from there.

30 Day Mucus Cleanse

Good for when there is a buildup of mucus or acidity through the body such as sinus, muscle acids, joint problems or respiratory weaknesses. Morning (M), Afternoon (A), Evening (E) Nature's Sunshine products (NSP)***Please see last page for NSP contact info.***

Cascara Sagrada: 1(M) 1(A) 2(E)

Psyllium: 2(M) 2(A) 2(E) open caps

Marshmallow & Pepsin: 2(M) 2(A) 2(E) open caps

Marshmallow & Fenugreek: 2(M) 2(A) 2(E) open caps

Bentonite Clay: 1 Tbsp. 3x between meals

Add if: sinus complaints – Sinus Support 2(M) 2(A) 2(E)

Joint pain – Bone & Skin Poultice 2(M) 2(A) 2(E)

Muscle Aches – Safflower 2(M) 2(A) 2(E)

Sinus Support, Bone & Skin, Marshmallow & Pepsin, Marshmallow & Fenugreek are NSP

First Time Cleansers

Tiao He Cleanse

Cleanses the liver and intestines. It is mild, adjustable and can be used on a monthly basis. Beginners: 1 of each 2x a day, 3 weeks on, 1-2 weeks off. Repeat, repeat. Experienced users: 1 of each 2x/day, 1 month on, 1 week off. Repeat, repeat.

Chinese Liver Balance (Nature's Sunshine Product- NSP)

All Cell Detox (NSP) capsules

LBSII (NSP) capsules

Psyllium Hulls capsules

Burdock capsules

Black Walnut capsules

Busy People on the Go

Ivy's Cleanse

May be taken on a daily basis. Keeps colon toned; good long-term results. Beginners: 1x per day, 3 weeks on, 1 to 2 weeks off. Repeat, repeat. Experienced users: 1x per day, 1 month on, 1 week off. Repeat, repeat.

2 Tbsp. liquid Chlorophyll

2 Tbsp. Aloe Vera Juice

1 tsp. Psyllium Hulls

2 Cascara Sagrada capsules

Mix and take first 3 ingredients with apple or other unfiltered juice then take Cascara with at least 8oz of water.

17 Day Deep Cleanse

Intestinal cleanse to scrape walls, clean out pockets and remove worms/mucus. Can be used every 2 to 3 months. Beginners: 2 of each 1-2x per day – 3 weeks. Experienced: 2 of each 3 times per day – 4 weeks.

Cascara Sagarada capsules

Psyllium Hulls capsules

Black Walnut capsules

All Cell Detox (NSP) capsules

Liver Cleanse Formula (NSP) capsules

2 Day Liver/Gallbladder Flush

For 5 or more days eat light and drink pure unfiltered apple juice and one of the following items: Stone Root, Gravel Root or Hydrangea (take recommended serving)

Day following above, fast for the next 2 days during flush:

Day 1
14 hydrangea capsules – 7 (M), 7(E) -NSP
6 Gallbladder Formula – NSP

Apple juice (diluted 50/50), water, and

lemon juice (may mix all three)

Day 2
Same as Day 1, plus
At bedtime, ½ C. squeezed lemon juice, ½ C. cold

pressed olive oil. Mix, drink and go right to bed,

lay on right side.

Next morn, be prepared to pass what looks like green peas.   These are gallstones. Drink plenty of liquids and break the fast with light foods. If nothing is passed, repeat at another time.   The Seneca Indian Fast would be good before this Flush, especially if nothing happens the first time.

Parasite Cleanse

Rids the body of fungus and parasites. May need to be repeated 10 days on and 10 days off at least 3 times – start near time of the full moon.

In order of importance:

Para free – 1 dropper 3x/day (Young Living)

Artemisia (Mugwort herb) - two 3x/day

Herbal Pumpkin – two 3x/day (NSP)

Black Walnut – two 3x/day

Caprylic Acid – two 3x/day

Cascara or LB formula – one 3x/day

Garlic – one 2x/day (morning & evening)

Black Currant oil – one 2x/day (morning & evening)

Anti-Pesticide/Herbicide/Fungicide Cleansing Tea

Herbal tinctures may also be substituted for dried herbs. Blend equal parts of each and steep 1 teaspoon of blend to 1 cup of hot water.

Burdock Root

Red Clover

Lemon Verbena

Ginger

Anti-Plastic (zenoestrogens) Cleansing Tea

Herbal tinctures may also be substituted. Blend equal parts of each and steep 1 teaspoon of blend to 1 cup of hot water.

Fenugreek

Mullein

Lemon Balm

Olive Leaf

Cottage Cheese Formula

This comes from Dr. Johanna Budwig. The cottage cheese and oil helps the body in producing interferons, which fights against viruses and tumors.

- 2 Cups organic cottage cheese
- 4 Tbsp. cold pressed walnut, almond, flaxseed or apricot oil

Mix together and eat all of it every day for two weeks. This is a foundation recipe. A variety of other ingredients such grated horseradish, chives, onions, parsley, cilantro, radishes (leaves and root), chopped spinach, kale or other greens may be added. (Budwig, 2017)

CONDITIONS

Herbal remedies have been used for thousands of years, for many types of conditions. When considering using these wonderful plants given to use by God for our health, we must not approach them from our modern-day medical way of thinking. Treating the symptom and this herb for that condition does not help in the long run.

The primary consideration when conditions present themselves is the root cause. Then the herb or herbs that can assist the body with the source of the issue may be applied. By dealing with the source, the body is able to bring itself back to homeostasis and thus, effect whatever the said condition. Of course, proper nutrition, elimination of toxins, conventional drugs being taken, the person's commitment to truly becoming well, etc., plays a vital part in the outcome.

Besides the root cause, another important consideration is the innate constitutions of herbs (energetics). Are they cooling, warming, hot or cold? For instance, cayenne has a hot constitution. It will warm you up, even make some too hot and open the sinuses as well. The same is also considered for the potential client. Each person also has an innate core body temperature; it tends to run too warm or too cool. For example, in general, if a person always needs a sweater, etc. to stay warm, even when the surrounding atmosphere is pleasant, then they are possibly a cold constitution person. Some herbs are of neutral constitution and has neither a hot or cold effect. There are other factors that may be playing a role that could present a false constitution which is why one should see their natural health practitioner for a health evaluation before addressing serious conditions.

Acid Reflux

Acidic gastric fluid from the stomach backs up into the esophagus, which causes heartburn. Also known as GERD (gastroesophageal reflux disease).

Potential Cause(s)

The conventional thought is too much acid in the stomach, but there can also be too little as well. Hiatal hernia is also a cause to take into consideration. The Helicobacter pylori bacteria (H. pylori) can cause an infection, which is often associated with hiatal hernias. Genetically modified foods (GMOs) can also be another cause to look at. When the ileocecal valve (connection of the small intestines to the colon) does not close properly, it can be due to intestinal parasites, which will give this effect as well. (Carman, 2013)

Herbals

Instead of the common conventional way of dealing with this condition, let's see what is offered from nature:

Licorice root (*Glycyrrhiza spp.*) - A neutral herb with a sweet taste. It fortifies digestion, restores stomach lining and soothes pains and spasms in the stomach. This herb also possesses anti-inflammatory compounds. (Borrelli, 2000)

*Those with high blood pressure, should use Chinese licorice.

Slippery elm (*Ulmus fulva*) – This neutral herb is soothing to the digestive tract. In its powdered form, it is customarily used to relieve heartburn because of its protective film, making it very healing.

Ginger (*Zingiberis officinale*) – A warming and common herb, consumed by many in various ways. It is used by many for relieving nausea. As the saying goes, an apple a day, keeps the doctor away; so, a teaspoon of freshly grated ginger a day, keeps the reflux away. Research also shows that it helps to inhibit the growth of H. Pylori bacteria. (Mahady, 2003)

Anxiety

There are a variety of anxieties. It could range from nervousness over taking a test to obsessive compulsiveness, as well as stress from various traumatic events and socially related anxiety. Anxiety can manifest in many ways such as nightmares, worrying, insomnia, excessive sweating, panic, increased heart rate, just being afraid and even fainting.

Potential Cause(s)

There are some common causes that connects the various forms of nervous system disorders. Some of these are vitamin, minerals, and omega-3 deficiencies. Also, amino acid deficiencies which affects the neurotransmitters of the brain and blood sugar imbalances. Food sensitivities or allergies are also categories to look at.

Herbals

Besides counselors or therapists, prescriptions are often used to deal with these types of nervous system disorders, but let's see what is offered from nature:

Milky Oats (*Avena sativa*) –This is a neutral herb and in tincture form is very effective for anxiety issues. It is bursting with nutrients and is a good blood sugar balancer especially since the adrenals become very fatigued under such conditions. (Chatueved, 2011)

Passionflower (*Passiflora incarnate*) – This cooling herb is very successful for nervous tension, difficulty with sleep and heart palpitations. A very good choice for the timid personality type. (Speroni, 1988)

Colitis and Crohns

These conditions afflict many today. Chronic inflammation and ulceration of the colon and rectum lining describes Colitis. Diarrhea with blood are symptoms of this condition which can be very painful. Crohns is a very severe form of Colitis and can extend from the mouth to the anus, but is mostly prominent at the end of the ileum (the third/

lower portion of the small intestines).

<u>Potential Cause(s)</u>

The causes of this type of bowel inflammation is usually connected to some type of infection, autoimmune issue, lack of blood supply to that area of the body, but often, food sensitivity or food allergies are at the root as well as GMOs.

<u>Herbals</u>

Marshmallow root (*Althaea officinalis*) – This cooling herb is very soothing to the irritated bowels. It has a slippery texture which coats the inner lining the mucous membranes of the intestines to reduce further damage. According to research, it is the most anti-inflammatory of the common mucilages." (Wood, 2008)

Turmeric (*Curcuma longa*) – Inflammation weakens the intestines barrier function, leading to its permeability. This hot herb's astringent qualities tighten and tones the intestinal wall as well as suppresses inflammation within the gastrointestinal tract. Turmeric also aids in health gut flora. (Baliga, 2012)

Cysts and Fibroids of the Breast and Uterus

Cysts are usually sac filled with fluid, pus, gas or semi-solid substance. They are usually noncancerous, but can be painful depending on size and location. Fibroids are solid tumors made up of fibrous connective tissue and smooth muscle cells. They are also known as myomas, fibromas and leiomyomas.

Potential Cause(s)

These types of growths are signs of imbalances in the hormonal system. Substances that imitate estrogen (synthetic or natural), causing an imbalance in function of the endocrine system. Pharmaceuticals estrogen therapy is also one of the culprits. The liver will often become congested due to working hard to remove these from the body.

Parasitic infection can also be a cause. If the lymphatic system is not moving sufficiently to remove toxicity, problems can also develop. There may also be a connection to an iodine or potassium deficiency which should be looked into.

Herbals

Maca root (*Lepidium meyenii*) – is a cooling herb that has been used traditionally, especially by the women of Peru and shown to be a very powerful tonic for the endocrine system. Clinical studies in Peru have suggested uterine fibroids have dissolved in just a few months in native women using it as supplementation. (Chacon, 1961)

Chickweed (*Stellaria media*) – is wonderful at cooling inflamed tissues which helps the lymph move and supports the body in dissolving cysts and tumors. Matthew Wood said, "...chickweed acts deeply on the body, decongesting the lymphatics and clearing waters through the kidneys driving off local pockets of water in the lungs or elsewhere, but also preserving and balancing the water levels in the body. In short, there is no area in the "alterative category" (liver, lymphatics, lungs) it does not touch." (Wood, 472)

Kidney stones

Solidified calcium oxalate or calcium phosphate and uric acid in the kidneys are known as kidney stones. These form over time and can be as small as a grain of sand to larger than a golf ball. There can be no symptoms to agonizing pain. They can cause urinary damage depending on their size and if they get lodged in the tubes of the urethra, leading to inflammation and infection.

<u>Potential Cause(s)</u>

The main cause is lack of enough water. Also, excessive acidity from such things as calcium supplements, processed foods and sugar; in addition, oxalates from chocolate, coffee and tanning-rich teas.

<u>Herbals</u>

Gravel Root (*Eupatorium purpureum*) - It is traditionally used stones in the kidneys. It has both diuretic and anti-lithic properties (acting against formation of calculi). It encourages an increase in urine and solid particles, supporting excretion of excess uric acid.

Hydrangea Root (*Hydrangea Arborescens*) - This cooling herb also has anti-lithic properties and helps the body to remove stones. It is said to coat the crystalized stones for easy passage. It has also been known to work within days in severe cases.

Prostatitis

One of the common issues with males as they get older, especially after 40 years, is the benign enlargement of the prostate. Due to this enlargement, the urethra narrows leading to various urinary problems. Such issues as urgency to urinate, feeling of unemptied bladder, dripping after and between urinating, painful urination and increase in frequency of urination.

Potential Cause(s)

Some possible reasons why the prostate may become enlarged are overproduction of dihydrotestosterone (DHT), a hormone metabolite, viral infections, sexually transmitted infections such as Chlamydia, and bacterial infections such as Staphylococcus or E. coli.

Herbals

Pumpkin Seed (*Cucurbita pepo*) - is a cooling herb that has been used in its raw form for centuries as a preventative for this type of issue. This is due to its DHT-blocking effects as well as several other plant steroids. (Heeok, 2009)

Saw Palmetto (*Serenoa repens*) – This is a widely known herb for its benefits to the prostate. From extensive studies, it is reported to also block DHT. Estrogen and progesterone are hormones involved with the production of DHT and Saw Palmetto is believed to reduce excessive production of these hormones. (Pais, 2010)

Cancer

One of the main principles of natural health is the whole person approach, regardless of condition; because a specific type of cancer is present, does not negate this principle, but makes it more vital. This kind of imbalance in the body is a systemic one and every area must be addressed. Anyone suffering from this condition should consider incorporating the Cottage Cheese Formula into the diet.

Potential Cause(s)

There are various reasons for the multiple types of cancers that plague society today. Dietary habits play a significant role in many cancers; research shows that sugar feeds cancer. Another powerful link to cancer shown in research is emotional shocks and traumas that are connected to the location and type of cancer.

Herbals

Sweet Violet (*Viola odorata L.*) – is well

known for use in addressing tumors (breast, intestines, lung and throat). (Mills, 500)

Has been used to treat skin cancer using the leaves as poultice as far back as 500 BC.

Cleavers (*Galium aparine*) – is able to detoxify various elimination pathways in the body at the same time due to its diaphoretic, diuretic, and mild laxative properties.

HAPPY CLEANSING :)

BIBLIOGRAPHY

Aguirre, N., Dr. and Baker, B., Dr. *Herbology Science and Forms of Cleansing.* Naturopathic Institute of Therapies & Education, 2016.

Baliga, M.S., Fayad, R., Joseph, N., Ponemone, V., Saxena, A., Venkataranganna, M.V., *Curcumin, an active component of turmeric in the prevention and treatment of ulcerative colitis: preclinical and clinical observations.* Food Funct. 2012 Nov; 3(11);1109-17. doi: 10. 1039/c2fo30097d.

Borrelli F and Izzo AA. *The Plant Kingdom as a Source of Anti-Ulcer Remedies.* Phytother Res. 2000; 14: 581-591., www.sciepub.com/reference/143906.

Burroughs, Stanley. *Healing for the Age of Enlightenment: Balanced Nutrition, Vita Flex, Color Therapy.* Burroughs Books, 1993.

Carman, J.A., Clinch-Jones, C.A., Edwards, J.W., Haynes, J.I., Robinson, G.W., Sneller,

V.E., Ver Steeg, L.J., Vlieger, H.R. 2013. *A long-term toxicology study on pigs fed a combined genetically modified (GM) soy and GM maize diet.* Journal of Organic Systems 8(1):38-54.

Chacon, G. *Pytochemical study on Lepidium meyenii.* PhD Thesis. Universidad Nacional Mayor de San Marcos. Lima, Peru. 1961, 1-46.

Chatueved, N., Shukla, K., Yadav, C.S. Diversified therapeutic potential of *Avena sative: An exhaustive review.* Pelagia Research Library. Asian Journal of Plant Science and Research, 1(3), 2011, 103-114.

Hong, H., Kim, C., Maeng, S., *Effects of pumpkin seed oil and saw palmetto oil in Korean men with symptomatic benign prostatic hyperplasia.* Nutr Res Pract. 2009 Winter; 3(4): 323-327.

Mahady, G.B.1, Pendland, S.L., Yun, G.S., Lu, Z.Z., Stoia, A., *Ginger (Zingiber officinale Roscoe) and the gingerols inhibit the growth of Cag A+ strains of Helicobacter pylori,* Anticancer Res. 2003 Sep-Oct; 23(5A);

3699-702.

Mills, Simon. *Out of the Earth: The Essential Book of Herbal Medicine.* Viking Penguin, 1991.

Minghetti, A., Speroni, E. Neuropharmacological Activity of Extracts from *Passiflora incarnate. Planta Medica.* 54; 488-491, 1988.

"The Budwig Diet – Flaxseed Oil and Cottage Cheese." *Cancer Tutor,* 24 July 2017, www.cancertutor.com/budwig/.

Wood, M., *The Earthwise Herbal: A Complete Guide to Old World Medicinal Plants.* North Atlantic Books, 2008.

C

F

H

I

K

L

S

T

U

V

JENNISE CANNON

Cancer, 3, 13

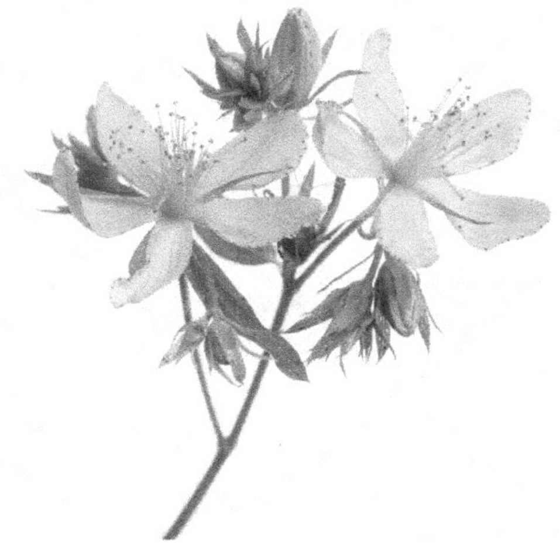

Wholistic Everyday Health, LLC
Jennise Cannon, N.D.
989.501.2343

wholisticeverydayhealth@protonmail.com